Sleep

Easy Sleep Solutions: 74 Best Tips for Better Sleep Health: How to Deal With Sleep Deprivation Issues Without Drugs Book

By Chris A. Baird

Sleep: Easy Sleep Solutions: 74 Best Tips for Better Sleep Health: How to Deal With Sleep Deprivation Issues Without Drugs Book

Table of Contents

1 - Introduction

This book is the fourth book in the bestselling PowerLists™ book series. Each PowerList™ book is designed to help you get more out of life.

Why Did I Write This Book?

I wrote this book because sleep is often overlooked despite its important role in our lives. Many people struggle or fail to get enough sleep. I hope that my book will equip you with the tools you need to get more sleep whether the reason is sleep deprivation or because you aren't making sleep a priority.

How To Use This Book

It is impossible for anyone to implement all of the suggestions I have in this book. However, if my tips help you sleep more and also get more out of your sleep, I will have succeeded in the purpose of this book. Try out the different tips and see what does or doesn't work for you.

Easy Sleep Solutions Cheat Sheet

I created a two page pdf *Easy Sleep Solutions Cheat Sheet*[1] to make it easy for you to be able to follow along as you work through the book. It shows you all 74 Tips and Tricks and can be used as a checklist or refresher on the different methods explored in the book.

---

[1] http://www.powerlists.org/7v84

2 - What Is Sleep?

"Sleep is that golden chain that ties health and our bodies together." - Thomas Dekker

"Sleep: the natural state of rest during which your eyes are closed and you become unconscious." - <u>Sleep</u>[2] . *Merriam-Webster Dictionary.*

These definitions give us a basic idea of what sleep is. However, if we are going to learn how to get better sleep, we need to do more than shut our eyes and go unconscious.

Misconceptions

"Until the 1950s, most people thought of sleep as a passive, dormant part of our daily lives. We now know that our brains are very active during sleep." - "<u>What is Sleep?</u>[3] " *American Sleep Association (ASA).*

A good place to start is to see what sleep isn't. As the ASA points out, it's not just the time of day where we do nothing. They thought it was just a period to give the brain a break. However, advances in neuroscience have shown that our

---

[2]http://www.powerlists.org/2ev2

[3]http://www.powerlists.org/vzmb

brains aren't taking breaks at all.

How Much Sleep Is Necessary

Although it varies from person to person, "most healthy adults need between seven and a half to nine hours of sleep per night to work at their best. Children and teens need even more." - "How Much Sleep Do You Need?[4] " *Help-Guide.org*.

Children need 12-18 hours of sleep and the numbers drop to 7.5-9 after the age of 18. The quantity of sleep that teen-agers and preteens get has decreased because of the impact of technology.

Later in the book, we will discuss the consequences.

____

[4]http://www.powerlists.org/ngwe

3 - Stages of Sleep

We are going to look under the hood of how sleep works. We will need to understand that there are different types of sleep. By understanding the stages of sleep, you will see how your choices impact these stages.

As you sleep, you pass through 5 stages. These include stages 1, 2, 3, 4 and Rapid Eye Movement (REM). You will move through the 5 stages in anywhere from 90-110 minutes. Once you have finished REM, you will then return for another cycle of sleep and repeat the 5 stages.

Stage 1

This is the stage when you are falling asleep. It is the border between being awake and being asleep. It is characterized by a light form of sleep. Your eyes will move slowly.

During this stage some people sense their muscles tighten and experience the sensation of falling. I experience this several times a year. You experience the sense of your body falling when you are partly awake and then become fully awake.

Stage 2

This is the stage where you start falling asleep and disconnect with the outside world. Your breathing rate and heart rhythm take on regular patterns and your body temperature drops. Your heart rate also slows down.

Another sign of this stage is that your eye movement stops. In addition, your brain waves slow down except for now and then when they spike. This stage accounts for 50% of your total sleep time.

Stage 3

This is where deep sleep kicks in. Both Stages 3 and 4 are called deep sleep. During this stage, it is difficult to wake a person. When you wake a person in Stage 3, they are disconnected from reality and it takes time for the world to become clear and for them to feel connected again.

It is during this deep sleep that the "body repairs and regrows tissues, builds bone and muscle tissue, and strengthens the immune system." - Jennifer Robinson, MD. - "What Are REM and Non-REM Sleep?[5] " *Webmd.*

---

[5]http://www.powerlists.org/hzaf

You should pay close attention to what is happening here. This is where lack of sleep prevents vital maintenance of the body.

Stage 4

In the United States, stages 3 and 4 are called Stage 3. However, elsewhere in the world, Stage 4 is known for being the stage where the brain produces mostly delta waves. These are the waves seen in the brain as the electrical activity in the brain oscillates between 1-8 Hz during sleep.

Sleep walking, nightmares, and even bed wetting for children occur during Stages 3 and 4.

REM

This stage of sleep is characterized by eye movement and dreaming.

This stage of sleep kicks in around 90 minutes after falling asleep. The first time you go into REM sleep, it will last 10 minutes. For each additional cycle, you will see an increase in REM sleep. It may reach as long as an hour and unlike the other stages, you will breathe faster and have an increased heart rate.

During REM sleep, your body loses the ability to regulate its temperature. That means that if your body is cold or hot based upon the external environment, you can be pulled out of REM sleep. However, your body will then allow you to slip back into REM sleep to ensure that you complete that part of the cycle. This stage of sleep accounts for 20% of your total sleep time.

REM sleep is important for learning since it stimulates the areas of the brain used in learning. Experiments have shown the effect when people are taught a skill and then deprived of REM sleep. They lose the ability to recall the skill when compared to people who are allowed to have REM sleep. Thus, of all the stages of sleep, REM is the most important for learning.

Circadian Rhythms

Circadian rhythms are the physical and mental changes that happen throughout the day. Try to think about them as a biological clock. This clock governs when a person is awake and when a person is tired. The natural cycle for a person deprived of light is 25 hours, during which a person moves between sleeping and being awake.

A blind person often has permanent sleep problems because lack of light confuses their schedule. This condition is similar to what people experience from jet lag. They go on a trip across multiple time zones, but their bodies are still stuck in the previous time zone. Shift workers also face this challenge. They are working and sleeping on cycles that differ from the normal daily rotation.

Several therapies can help. Melatonin supplements help stabilize the daily circadian rhythm. Another option is using bright lights--much brighter than normal lights--when trying to train oneself to wake up.

Technology for Tracking Sleep Cycles

The market is now filled with apps for the iPhone and Android that can track sleep cycles. Based upon your movement, sounds, and breathing, it is possible to deduce where you are in the sleep cycle. A graph will show how long the cycles are lasting and the app will make recommendations for improvement.

4 - Signs You Aren't Getting Enough Sleep

The easiest way to tell if you aren't getting enough sleep is to see how you feel throughout the day. To complicate the matter, it's difficult to know how much sleep you are lacking when you are sleep deprived.

One reason it is so hard to notice the sleep deprivation is because it has become normal for you. By reviewing the signs of sleep deprivation, you will be better equipped to judge whether you suffer from this. None of these items alone mean you are sleep deprived, but they are indicators you may have a problem.

You Need to Sleep in on Weekends

The reason a person is exhausted on the weekend is because they haven't been getting enough sleep during weekdays. Their bodies attempt to compensate for the shortage of sleep. In fact, it isn't possible to compensate for that lack of sleep, but the body will try to compensate for it.

You Fall Asleep at Once When You Go to Bed at Night

A person who is exhausted or sleep deprived will fall asleep at once. There are exceptions for this rule as well. I am one of them since I always fall asleep within five minutes and I am not sleep deprived.

Getting Out of Bed in the Morning Is a Challenge

Do you find it difficult to get out of bed each morning? If so, this may indicate that you aren't getting enough sleep. I read about a celebrity who didn't use an alarm clock. Instead, she went to bed each night at a specific time knowing she would wake up at the right time in the morning.

If you are sleeping enough hours, it should be easy to wake up every day. You aren't trying to force yourself to sleep. Your body wakes up once it has the right amount of sleep. The problem is that when you are used to being sleep deprived, you assume that tiredness is normal.

You Hit the Snooze Button

This used to be a major problem for me in college. I remember my roommate and I took turns hitting the snooze button. We were sleep deprived, staying up late studying or socializing and being dead tired the next morning. Why do you need to hit the snooze button? The additional sleep isn't deep enough to leave you well rested, and it is a perfect sign that your body isn't getting the sleep you need.

You Have to Take a Nap in the Daytime

Taking a nap in the middle of the day for many people is a normal part of life. However, it reflects on your not getting enough sleep the night before. The nap itself will throw off your evening sleep schedule. The goal should be to sleep enough at night so that you are rested and can make it through the day.

You Fall Asleep During Classes at School or Meetings at Work

Falling asleep during class or meetings is another sign of sleep deprivation. In the military, I heard about a commander who slept only four hours each night. He dozed off in the middle of meetings. It left people wondering whether they should continue the meeting or first wake him up.

There is one reason you are falling asleep during these points in the day. That is because you aren't getting enough sleep the night before. There are exceptions to the rule; you should determine whether you are an exception or if you are lacking sleep.

You Doze Off in the Evening While Watching TV or Relaxing

The final category is falling asleep at the end of the day. It makes sense you may be tired after a long, hard day. However, you shouldn't be so dead tired that you cannot stay awake when watching TV or reading before bedtime. This is another sign of sleep deprivation.

Are You Sleep Deprived?

If you answered *yes* to one or more items on this list, you may be sleep deprived. One easy way to find out is to get more sleep and see if the signs go away. A person getting nine hours of sleep at night is far less likely to find it difficult to get up or to need to hit the snooze button.

They are unlikely to fall asleep during classes or meetings. The important thing to remember is that sleep deprivation comes at a price. It is worth exploring whether or not you are getting the right quantity of sleep.

5 - Myths About Sleep

Several myths surround sleep. By being aware of them, you won't fall into the trap of believing these false ideas about how to get better sleep.

It's Easy to Adjust to Changes in Your Sleep Schedule

Some people think that it doesn't matter when you go to bed or wake up. Maybe you stay up extra hours one night and get up early the next day. Or you mix it up and go to bed early and sleep in late. One myth says that you can easily adjust sleep patterns and schedules.

However, this is false. You are impacted by changes in your sleep schedule. By mixing up the times for sleeping and waking, you are confusing your brain.

Sleep Is Where the Body and Brain Do Nothing

"Until the 1950s, most people thought of sleep as a passive, dormant part of our daily lives." - "Brain Basics: Understanding Sleep[6] ." *National Institution of Neurolo-*

[6]http://www.powerlists.org/63fj

gical Disorders and Stroke (NINDS).

We have since learned that our brains are active during sleep. One of the key issues is that according to the NINDS:

"Research also suggests that a chemical called adenosine builds up in our blood while we are awake and causes drowsiness. This chemical breaks down while we sleep."

This means that a lack of sleep will prevent a person from the proper breakdown of this chemical. Thus, they begin the next day tired.

The reason this myth is bad is because it can lead people to believe that sleep isn't important that it is a time to relax and nothing else. It is easy to see why people might assume this. We appear to be doing nothing when we sleep. All the hormonal and brain activity is invisible unless we are watching the brain waves and chemicals during sleep.

Catching Up on the Weekend

A common myth says that sleeping on weekends will compensate for a shortage of sleep during the week. The problem is that it doesn't work this way.

No matter how much sleep you get on the weekend, your body can't compensate for the shortage of sleep. In addition, sleeping in late on the weekends throws off your sleep cycles, making getting up on Monday morning a greater challenge.

One or Two Hours Less Sleep Isn't a Big Deal

You may think that a loss of an hour or two of sleep isn't anything to worry about. People today sleep on average two hours less per night than people did in 1960.

Scientists at Cambridge, Harvard, Manchester and Surrey universities found that, "cancer, heart disease, type-2 diabetes, infections and obesity have all been linked to reduced sleep." - James Gallagher. "'Arrogance' of ignoring need for sleep[7]." *BBC*.

The amount of sleep deprivation required to trigger these negatives can be as little as a few hours a night. This should be taken seriously. The real issue here is whether you are getting enough sleep. If you aren't, a change is needed. This

---

[7]http://www.powerlists.org/su29

is true even if you lack only an hour each night.

6 - Consequences of Not Getting Enough Sleep

Many assume that not getting the right amount of sleep will mean being tired the next day but that with coffee you can compensate for the sleep or catch up on sleep later when you have more time.

The problem with that approach is that the consequences of sleep deprivation are huge. Let's explore what happens to you when you fail to get the minimum amount of required sleep.

Diabetes

A 2007 study published in the *Sleep Medicine Review* found that sleep deprivation triggers an increased risk of diabetes in multiple ways. This link can be difficult to draw since diabetes is connected to obesity. The fact is a shortage of sleep impacts the body's ability to handle glucose. This is an important point to note.

Lack of sleep triggers so many other problems. It is difficult to distinguish negative effects from sleep deprivation and the negative effects of triggers themselves. Whatever the case, by getting more sleep, you can decrease the various risks at the same time.

Heart Issues

Sleep plays an important role in reducing stress hormones in your system. Those hormones can damage your blood vessels and trigger high blood pressure or hypertension. High blood pressure can lead to heart disease and death.

This is an important lesson. If you want to have a healthy heart, you need to ensure you are getting enough sleep. That means *planning* to get more sleep. Your life may depend upon it.

Depression

The hormones that go out of balance when we lack sleep are involved with our energy and mood. When we get less sleep, we experience a negative change in mood. Some people get more sensitive and irritable. This may trigger us to be sad and overreact to negative circumstances in our environment. Depression is a high price to pay for doing something else instead of sleeping when we ought to.

Loss of Concentration

Our ability to concentrate decreases when the brain is tired from the night before. This means we will use more time to complete tasks at work and home. The quality of our work will be substandard. Clarity of thought and focus is most important when trying to get a task done quickly and accurately. When the brain is less focused, everything takes much more time.

Hallucinations

Another symptom of sleep deprivation is hallucinations. I can attest to having hallucinations. A long time ago, I was taking a trip. I had been driving for sixteen hours straight. Upon looking up, I saw a giant rabbit crossing the road. It jumped off the road before I got to it, but this was the first time I recall hallucinating.

In addition, I recall seeing lines on the road swerving as the hypnotic pattern of the reflectors on the road hit my eyes. I have since created a rule of not driving more than eight hours per day and never driving after 10 pm. Ignoring this rule could cost my life or someone else's.

Increase in Psychological Problems for Children

A Norwegian <u>study</u>[8] found that children with sleep issues sometimes later develop anxiety and depression problems.

It is difficult to know what triggers what. However, it is possible to say that there is a clustering of these issues. The best way to deal with these problems is for children to get adequate sleep.

Paranoia, Anxiety, and Irritability

People are often edgy when they are sleep deprived, and they perceive risks that aren't real; they are annoyed by their environment in a manner that is not normal.

Irritability is common when people are sleep deprived. Everything around them seems annoying. Sadness is common also. For this reason it is unwise to attempt problem solving when sleep deprived. It is best to postpone making big life decisions until sleep is regulated. This would also be true of telephoning people, sending email and texts.

---

[8]http://www.powerlists.org/7ya3

Skin Damage

As little as one night without sleep can lead to puffy eyes and skin issues. Chronic sleep deprivation can make these issues permanent. The elasticity of the skin can be damaged and lines on the face can remain even after you start getting sleep. The reason for this is that fatigue triggers the body to produce the hormone cortisol which breaks up the skin proteins responsible for keeping the skin elastic.

Inability to Learn

There are two ways in which sleep deprivation creates problems with learning:

- Impaired Short Term Memory

- Inability to Learn Even With Repetition

People who do not have adequate sleep experience impaired short term memories. This is seen in trying to recall things learned the day before. When a person isn't getting sleep, they struggle to remember.

Repeating a task will help a person remember. However, if

the person first does the task while sleep deprived, they will find it harder to remember that same task even with repetition. This is true even when the person has enough sleep the night before they attempt the task. When tired, the brain learn doesn't properly.

These two issues are important for students whose job is to learn and yet they often suffer sleep deprivation.

Forgetfulness

A lack of sleep will prevent you from learning new information. The problem doesn't stop there. This shortage of sleep affects your ability to remember what you have learned. People who are sleep deprived find they become much more forgetful than their peers who are getting the sleep they need.

Poor Decision Making

This consequence can be expensive. It is much easier to make poor decisions when sleep deprived. In fact, people become much more willing to take bigger risks when short on sleep.

Increased Sensitivity to Pain

People who experience a lack of sleep are much more aware of pain. This is a good reason for getting enough sleep. The opposite is also true. If you has are experiencing pain, getting more sleep will help you handle the pain.

Weight Gain

The body produces two hormones that are impacted by a lack of sleep. One is called leptin, which controls a person's appetite. The other hormone is ghrelin, which makes a person want to consume more food. A shortage of sleep, even a single night, is enough to cause a decrease in leptin and an increase in ghrelin. The result is that the person is hungry and will eat more.

"According to Clete Kushida, MD, PhD, RPSGT, a neurologist and sleep specialist at the Stanford Sleep Disorders Clinic in California. 'The more ghrelin you have, the more you want to eat.'" - "Not Enough Sleep: 7 Serious Health Risks[9]." *Webmd.*

---

[9] http://www.powerlists.org/car4

Weakened Immune System

If you aren't getting adequate sleep for as little as a single night, your immune system will lose its ability to fight off microorganisms. There is a connection between getting the appropriate quantity of sleep and your body's defense against bacteria and viruses.

Reduced Sex Drive

Men and women both experience a decrease in libido because of sleep deprivation. The body becomes exhausted, and the brain loses focus and desire. For men, there is a reduction in the testosterone levels triggering the drop in sex drive.

Headaches

Another common side-effect of sleep deprivation is headaches. The group hit the hardest are the people who already suffer from headaches. In particular, people who get migraine headaches can expect to increase the intensity and duration of their headaches when not getting enough sleep.

Drop in Reaction Time

Our ability to react to situations that demand our attention decreases with lack of sleep. This includes driving a car while tired. Many studies have shown the similarities between driving while intoxicated and driving while sleep deprived. The similarities are so close it should be illegal to drive when lacking sleep. The problem is the inability to test whether a person has had enough sleep the night before.

Death

Although this isn't common, it still makes the news every year when people die after staying awake for days playing video games. Sleep deprivation is a life threatening condition that should be taken seriously. Your life may depend upon how seriously you take it.

Problems with Vision

This problem can manifest itself in several ways, including dim vision, tunnel vision, or even double vision. It poses a risk when the person is driving a car or trying to accomplish something where vision is essential.

The Sum of Them All

One thing that should be clear is that the consequences of not getting enough sleep are terrible. The combination of these different issues creates a synergistic effect in amplifying the negatives.

It would be bad enough if these consequences hit you one at a time. That isn't how it works. Once you get into the habit of cutting your sleep short, you will experience several problems that trigger more problems. Sometimes it is difficult to figure out which problem is caused by lack of sleep since they all show up at the same time.

7 - Benefits of Sleep

Many of the benefits of sleep are the opposites of the consequences of not getting enough sleep. Though, if we want to change, we need to know why we ought to change. The advantages of getting enough sleep are so numerous that it is worth taking time with each.

Improved Driving

The last thing anyone wants is a car accident. By ensuring you are getting enough sleep, your reaction time improves and your overall driving ability will be at a much higher level. Driving is a life or death issue. So, getting your sleep can save yours or someone else's life.

Increased Productivity

People who sleep properly have a much higher level of focus and concentration than those who are sleep deprived. Their productivity is higher at work and home. It is difficult to focus on work and coordinate tasks when your brain is challenged.

Improved Learning Ability

Getting proper sleep will increase your ability to learn and remember what you have learned. The role of sleep is critical in the initial learning process and in later recalling that information. This is why it is especially important for children and students to get enough sleep.

Great for Losing Weight

The hormonal balancing that happens when we are asleep ensures that we don't feel hungry throughout the day. If you want to keep pounds off, getting a proper quantity of sleep will ensure greater success.

The opposite is true. If you overeat, you will not sleep well. The relationship between diet and sleep cannot be overstated. They both impact each other negatively or positively. If you can get one of them in order, it will impact the other positively.

Fewer Headaches

The number of headaches people experience drops when they get their necessary sleep. In particular, getting proper sleep reduces the number of migraines people experience. Not having headaches makes it easier to get to sleep.

This is the case for many of these situations. You deprive yourself of sleep and that triggers a consequence. Then, the consequence makes getting enough sleep difficult. It becomes a vicious cycle.

Better Muscle Building

Sleep plays an important role in the rebuilding of muscle after working out at the gym. Muscles are torn during the workout and need to be rebuilt. The repair of these torn muscles is something that everyone who wishes to build muscle mass needs to keep in mind.

Do You Want to Be Happier?

Sleep has a huge impact on your overall happiness and mood. Everything around us is more vivid and the negatives aren't as negative when we are well rested. Our overall outlook on life takes a positive turn when we add proper sleep to the picture.

Healthier Skin

People who get enough sleep have much better skin than those who don't. Skin damaged by ultraviolet light heals much faster for people who are sleeping well. This can account for increased aging in people who are sleep deprived.

You Speak Clearer

Another major advantage of getting enough sleep is that you will speak clearer. Those who are sleep deprived will:

- Slur words

- Speak in a monotone

- Speak slowly

- Repeat words

Young Adults Are Less Likely to Abuse Alcohol

Adolescents with a shortage of sleep have a higher rate of alcohol-related abuse than those who were sleeping properly. The abuse of alcohol impacts the quality of sleep.

A loop forms between the misuse of alcohol because of a lack of sleep and that same alcohol making it harder to sleep. In contrast, the young adults who had proper sleep had a much lower rate of abuse of alcohol.

8 - The Different Sleep Disorders

In America, 40 million people suffer from sleep disorders with another 20 million people having sleep difficulties from time to time.

The cost of these sleep issues results in medical costs of $16 billion each year. That may be much higher when indirect costs of sleep disorders are factored in.

"The most common sleep disorders include insomnia, sleep apnea, restless legs syndrome, and narcolepsy." - "<u>Brain Basics: Understanding Sleep</u>[10] ." *National Institution of Neurological Disorders and Stroke (NINDS).*

Insomnia

Insomnia is extremely common. It is something most people experience in life. It is most common as people get older, hitting 30 percent of men and 40 percent of women. There are a wide variety of triggers for insomnia including:

- Eating habits

- Jet-lag

------

[10]http://www.powerlists.org/s74p

- Stress

Sleep Walking

This problem can be hazardous if a person sleep walks to their car, to the stove, or into the street although for many, sleep walking lasts only 30 to 60 seconds. This issue happens during the REM stage of sleep and the person rarely remembers it the next day.

Snoring

Many people don't consider snoring to be a sleeping disorder; however, it is for several reasons. The top issue is that snoring creates noise which can interrupt your natural sleep cycle.

People assume that snoring will create issues for other people sharing your bed or room, Keep in mind that the sound in a room can be a problem. Snoring is not white noise that blends into the background.

Another issue related to snoring is that it may be a sign you are suffering from sleep apnea which we will explore later in this chapter. The key issue here is that a person isn't getting the oxygen they need. This leaves the person tired the next day. Even worse, not getting enough oxygen can lead to death if not treated. This is one important reason you should inform your doctor.

One way to find out if you are having a problem with snoring is to use an app on your phone like *Sleep Talk*. This app allows you to record your sleep at night. Then, you can listen to it the next day and see if you are having an issue with rolling around in the night or snoring. The app also records talking at night; however, it is great for recording snoring.

Nightmares

Nightmares happen during the REM stage of sleep. They disturb the ability to get a good night sleep and are triggered by drugs, stress, or anxiety. Most often they occur in children between the ages of three and five years old.

They may be helpful in identifying other issues in life that are triggering them. Anxiety and stress are issues that can cause poor sleep. If you throw in nightmares, you get a double negative.

The key issue with nightmares is figuring out what is triggering them. Then, dealing with the trigger can help decrease their frequency.

One trick I have used with children is I tell them to imagine that whatever is scary in the dream is a clown. That takes the edge off the nightmare. One time didn't work, ironically, when the nightmare was about a clown.

Tooth Grinding

Grinding your teeth can create sleep issues. Two that come to the forefront are:

- Headaches from the tightening

- The sounds produced

Both can wake you up or at least disturb your sleep cycles.

Many people experience this problem without knowing it. Damage to the teeth is a sure sign something is going on causing the teeth to be loose, worn, or chipped. If you have a partner, they may hear the sound from the grinding.

You should see your doctor if you are having this issue.

They can fit you with a mouth guard to use while sleeping which should prevent additional damage to your teeth and eliminate the sound at night.

Pregnancy

There are several issues that pregnancy brings to the forefront making sleep an issue. These include:

- Morning sickness (first trimester)

- Having to use the toilet often (first trimester)

- Back and other pains

- Vivid dreams

All of these issues are a normal part of being pregnant and can be more or less of a problem depending upon the person. Lack of sleep can trigger a host of other issues. Thus, it is important for pregnant women to stay in contact with their doctor and prioritize sleep for the sake of:

- The baby

- Your own health

Circadian Rhythm Disorders

These problems involve issues with your circadian rhythm being out of order. The word *circadian* itself is two words:

- "Circa" means "about"

- "Dies" means "day"

The circadian rhythm is the internal clock telling you about the day. The part of the brain that has this responsibility is the "suprachiasmatic nucleus." It attempts to keep you on a normal schedule of waking and sleeping.

There are several areas where you can experience problems with your circadian rhythm:

- Delayed Sleep Phase Syndrome - Falling asleep and waking up too late

- Advanced Sleep Phase Syndrome - Falling asleep and waking up too early

- Work Shift Changes - Switching work shifts

- Jet Lag - Traveling across time zones

In these situations, your internal clock is out of order. It isn't waking you up at the right time, nor is it telling you to go to sleep. In addition, even after falling asleep, your body may try to wake you up believing that it is morning or it may make it hard for you to fall asleep at all.

I have experienced falling asleep in the middle of the day when jet lagged. A day in the new time zone is required for each hour you have crossed over to readjust to a normal cycle. In some instances, the body fails to adjust leaving a person in a situation where sleep becomes a serious issue triggering other health issues.

Sleep Apnea

Sleep Apnea is a serious condition involving breathing disruption during asleep. Although there are exceptions, it is often associated with loud snoring. It is most common as a person grows older or has a fat buildup. As a result, the person may experience a collapse of the windpipe. In addition, the issue may be caused by the functioning of neurons which control breathing. The result is breaks in breathing.

Although many people struggle with sleep apnea, few see a specialist for the issue. The individual experiences a cycle of having their breathing stop and then they wake up and gasp for air. They get oxygen and fall back to sleep to repeat this cycle again.

This condition can be dangerous, and people who have the condition and take sleeping pills may not be able to wake up to catch a breath. Therefore, if you exhibit any of these symptoms, you should seek medical attention for a diagnosis.

The worst thing you can do is ignore the problem. It is possible to have this issue without realizing it. This is why the chapter on symptoms of sleep problems is important. If none of the tricks in this book work, you may need to see a doctor and be tested for sleep apnea.

Narcolepsy

The final disorder to be explored is narcolepsy. This is a condition that causes people to fall asleep at different times of the day. It can happen even when the person is well rested. In the late 90s, it was found that this condition is connected to a problem in the genes. It can be treated with regular naps and stimulants and even anti-depressants.

I mention the condition since it may tempt you to think of a person with the symptoms of narcolepsy as a sign of not getting enough sleep. However, that is incorrect. Being aware of different conditions can better help you find the treatment you need from your medical provider.

9 - Why Don't We Sleep More?

Failure to Recognize the Consequences

The top reason people don't get more sleep is because they don't believe there are consequences. In the preceding chapter we covered negative consequences and it should be clear now that ignoring sleep issues comes at a high price.

The best way to handle this problem is to look at the studies regarding the consequences and convince ourselves that this is too high a price to pay.

We Aren't Tired

There are a number of factors that keep us awake. They include easy access to entertainment including TV, cell phones, video games and computers. This, in part, involves exciting and engaging activities. In addition, the light from these devices and lights in our houses wake us up and trick us into thinking it is daytime.

Some people are night owls. This trait can be connected to drinking too much coffee too late in the day or to smoking. Whatever the case, not being tired is a major issue in exploring why we don't go to sleep.

We Have Too Much to Do

This reason is often connected to our work, but our hobbies can motivate us to feel so busy that we work late hours. Binge working or studying not effective. Our brains aren't working as well when we are sleep deprived and cramming keeps us from retaining that information.

We Want to Get More Out of the Day

People have a long list of things to do during the day. This is true particularly true when compared with people 25 years ago. There has been a drop in the amount of sleep people are getting and an increase in the urge to get more done. This pressure to do more results in less sleep.

There is irony in this, especially for people who get up early to exercise. The problem is that lack of sleep takes a toll on health even when they lose sleep in order to exercise. The exercise does not make up for loss of sleep.

10 - Why Not Use Sleeping Pills?

In today's over-medicated society, it is a myth to think that a few more pills should solve our problems. Sometimes it is necessary to take medication, and each person needs to consult their doctor.

I am not a doctor and have no intention of giving medical advice. What I intend is to point out what the research shows about using drugs to treat sleeping disorders. What you do with this information is an issue between you and your doctor.

Causing Insomnia

People who suffer from insomnia are often prescribed sleeping pills. However, in most cases sleeping pills quit working after a few weeks. In an even more odd twist, when taken over a long period of time sleeping pills can make sleeping problems worse.

Strange Side Effects

Sleeping pills can cause amnesia and sleep walking. People sometimes wake up and forget where they are. Sometimes a person assumes that the effect of the pills will take time so they don't go to bed right away. As the pills take effect, a person can go from being awake to a dreamlike state before they reach their bed.

Tired During the Day

Another issue is that sleeping pills can continue working even after you wake up the next day. This creates a huge problem if you are driving while still under the influence of these drugs. You may find yourself tired when trying to work the next day.

Loss of Balance

Sleeping pills can affect balance causing people to fall. This is an issue for older people especially.

Building up a Tolerance

A person who takes sleeping pills for more than two weeks will notice that the effect of the medication diminishes. This may cause people to increase the dose to achieve the same result; however, the other side effects increase with doses beyond the recommended daily amount.

Dependency on Pills

A person who continues taking sleeping pills over time will find that insomnia may happen the moment they attempt to stop taking them. This is one reason you may need to slowly decrease intake.

Mixing with Other Drugs

Taking sleeping pills and alcohol or stimulants will cause the effects of both drugs to be amplified. This means you may find yourself even more tired when you wake up. Sometimes people have had breathing problems requiring emergency treatment.

Use Them as a Last Resort

Sleeping pills deliver on their promise. They promise to get you to sleep and that is what they do. However, this comes at a cost as we have discussed. There are plenty of tricks and tips in this book that don't involve using drugs to fall asleep. If nothing is working, then sleeping pills may be right for you if your doctor sees no other option.

If you go this route, make sure you try them for a few weeks.

They should help correct a negative sleeping cycle and even build a habit of going to sleep at a specific time. It is important to take the recommended doses and watch for negative side effects.

Taken as a last resort and under a doctor's supervision, sleeping pills may help. However, considering all of the risks associated with these pills, you should first exhaust all other options.

11 - Tricks for Better Sleep

(1) Keep to a Schedule

Our minds and bodies follow daily patterns. If we train ourselves to do the same thing over and over, we will form habits. These habits prepare our body to perform the ritual or habit of going to sleep.

Many people make the mistake by changing the time they go to bed and wake up. This can include what they do on weekends.

A better solution is to choose a time of night you will go to sleep and a time you will wake up and stick to that schedule. On weekends, I sometimes stay up an extra hour and then get up an hour later.

Sticking to a schedule prepares your mind to follow the pattern. This is very similar to eating. You can train your body to have different expectations, and falling asleep becomes much easier. I explore the role of habits in my book *Habit Ignition: 41 Steps to Unlocking the Secret Power of Habits and Rituals for Life Book*[11] .

---

[11]http://www.powerlists.org/03k6

(2) Set Calming Activities for Your Bedtime Ritual

The key with this trick is that we are creatures of habit. Establish a habit of doing calming activities every night before bed. They will train your brain to associate those activities with falling asleep.

A few of these activities include:

- Take a warm bath

- Drink a warm cup of milk or decaffeinated tea

- Do a favorite hobby (not an exciting one)

- Listen to an audio book

- Stretch (light stretching only)

- Listen to soft music

- Prepare things for the next day

- Read a book or magazine under a gentle light

(3) Let There Be Darkness

The brain contains a structure called the suprachiasmatic nucleus (SCN) which contains 20,000 neurons. The SCN sends signals to the pineal gland which responds to light by switching on and off the production of the hormone melatonin. When it is dark, the production of melatonin increases which makes a person tired. If a person is exposed to light, the melatonin won't decrease and the person won't feel tired.

Therefore, the best environment for sleeping is complete darkness. This can be difficult to achieve because light comes from windows, mobile phones, or alarm clocks.

You can solve this problem by ensuring that all light is blocked out. You can buy light-blocking plastic curtains that will block 100% of the light from entering your room from the outside.

The next challenge is technology. I have found great success putting light-blocking covers over all devices. My cell phone is turned upside down to prevent it from shooting light at me. Previously my alarm was a standard digital alarm clock until I learned this trick.

Even the glowing red light of an alarm clock is enough to disturb your sleep. So, when we say the trick is to have no light, we mean no light. It should be pitch black in your room.

In the far north of Norway, people who grew up with the midnight sun have adjusted to it. Others have found that putting aluminum foil over the windows helps block out all light. By looking at dorm windows at the university, you can tell which rooms house people who aren't natives of the North; there is foil on those windows.

This specific trick is so important I will look for even the faintest glow of light coming into the bedroom and ensure that it is removed.

Children sometimes use nightlights to cope with darkness. However, darkness is the best environment for them. They won't sleep as well with light in their rooms. We have to find a compromise on this issue. So, the goal should be to have as little light as possible.

(4) Use Eye Masks

Eye masks are cheap and you can put them over your eyes to block out the light. Keep in mind that not all blinders are equal. Some are made of thin cloth material whereas the ones made of foam are much better at ensuring that no light gets through them.

I find, in Norway, the light is so bright early in the morning I have to find a better solution when spending the night at local cabins. The eye blinders make it difficult to fall asleep so I put them on when I am first awakened by the light. Then, I can sleep till my normal wake-up time with them in place. This was a real game changer for me and could be for you.

(5) Sleep in Different Bed Than Your Partner

One in four couples in the United States reported sleeping in separate beds than their partners. A phrase used to describe this is a "sleep divorce." People should be able to sleep in the same bed; however, if your partner's sleep habits of snoring, talking, or rolling around is leaving you restless, you should sleep in different beds or rooms.

There is a possibility that your partner may be the cause your sleep issues. The consequences of not getting enough sleep will impact your relationship.

It is strange that a great way to improve your relationship with your partner is to sleep apart. They shouldn't abandon you or cut out other activities. It may be a good idea to move to a different room right before you plan to go to sleep.

Like most tricks, this may not be the first trick you try for better sleep. However, the consequences of sleep deprivation are so huge that you need to consider whatever is necessary to get your sleep in order. That can help your relationship.

(6) No Screens Before Bed

"Research has shown that blue light keeps you awake because it suppresses the production of melatonin." - Kelly Oakes. "14 Scientific Hacks To Help You Get a Better Night's Sleep[12] ." *Buzzfeed.*

---

[12]http://www.powerlists.org/q86k

The problem with the modern world is that we are looking at screens. This includes TVs, computers, and smartphones. Our bodies are built to use the light outside to signal whether it is day or night.

The suppression of melatonin confuses our bodies and makes us think that it is day when it is night. This is bad news for us if we hope that falling asleep will be easy. It is like trying to catch up on sleep in the middle of the day with the sun overhead. It is possible but requires more work since our brain tells us it is day.

This is a problem for children here in Norway. They think it is day late into the night since the sun is still visible in the sky. It is hard to convince them to go back to sleep when they see light outside and their brains tell them it is still day. The same goes for early in the morning.

The opposite happens in the winter time when it is dark all of the time. It's hard to get up when it is pitch black outside, but sleeping is easier when it is dark.

The solution is tough to implement. Avoid looking at your smartphones and other devices an hour or two prior to bed-time. I know this one is hard; my phone is what I look at right before bed. If sleep is a problem, then, as Sir Otto Lilienthal said, "Sacrifices must be made."

Another option you can try is using glasses to block out blue light. A study[13] done on the use of these glasses showed that people using these glasses got just as much sleep as people in complete darkness.

(7) Don't Change Your Schedule Even When Sleep Deprived

When you fail to get enough sleep the night before, you may be tempted to go to bed early the next night to compensate. The problem is that you will change your overall schedule. A better solution is to stay with your current schedule. Following a schedule is the best way to train the body to go to sleep at a specific time.

If you stay up late one night and get up at your normal time, you can expect to be tired. When you go to sleep the next night you can expect to be extra tired. It is important to keep repeating the behavior until your body surrenders and falls asleep at the scheduled time.

----

[13]http://www.powerlists.org/cbid

(8) Don't Wait Until You Are Sleepy

It is important to listen to your body. However, this isn't always the case. For sleep and setting a routine, you may or may not be sleepy when it is time for bed. I often get a burst of energy right before bed. I want to stay up many hours beyond my bedtime. It is a terrible idea to wait until I am tired. It is best to go to bed at the scheduled time whether you are tired or not.

In the worst case scenario, you are unsuccessful at falling asleep. You get up and do something else until you get tired. I can often fall asleep even if I don't feel tired.

Part of controlling the environment and the routine is to force you to be tired. If your bedroom is associated with sleep, going into the room pulls a psychological trigger. Therefore, you shouldn't use your sleepiness as a way of determining if it is time to go to sleep.

(9) Avoid Drinking Liquids Two Hours Before Bed

If we have a problem with falling asleep, having to use the

toilet will not make the situation better. Instead, we need to focus on ways of keeping ourselves in bed throughout the night. It is best to avoid drinking liquids during the two-hour period before going to bed.

Following this tip is an effective way to ensure that all of the liquid in your system is processed prior to trying to go to sleep. Thus, you will stay in bed the entire night without having to get up to use the toilet.

Many of these tips follow a pattern. It is all about keeping yourself in bed with as few disruptions as possible. If you want to get better sleep, get rid of anything and everything that disturbs your sleep.

(10) Slow Down Your Breathing

It is helpful to slow your breathing when you are trying to get your brain to stop focusing on the chaos from a day. And you need to avoid planning for the next day. By breathing in through your nose and out through your mouth you find that your brain calms down.

Even during daytime hours when I need to calm down, this exercise can be very effective. Many times I will fall asleep doing deep breathing exercises. I do a rotation of 7 breaths per minute to get the full effect of filling my lungs and then emptying them. The goal isn't to experience pain. Rather, you need to maximize the sensation of fullness and emptiness in the lungs.

(11) Replace Your Pillow Every 12 to 18 Months

Many people assume that their pillows last forever. In fact, they last a year to two before they should be swapped out. This is true for several reasons:

- Dust Mites

- Head Support

I am allergic to dust mites and the bed is a place where they build up. By swapping out your pillow, you ensure you don't trigger an allergic reaction to these pests.

The second reason is equally important. Just like our mattresses, our pillows provide support for us while we sleep. After a while, a pillow loses its form and no longer does a good job of supporting the head. Thus, it is important to swap out the pillow before it reaches this point. You can identify when it is time by noticing stiffness in your head, neck and back in the morning.

Another thing to consider is that you should choose a pillow based upon how you sleep. Different pillows work best for people who sleep on their side, back, or belly. On the firmness front, side-sleeping people need a firm pillow. Get a new pillow every year or two.

(12) Keep Your Room Clean

There is a connection between clutter and stress levels. By keeping the room clean and orderly, you will reduce your stress and thus be removing another trigger that is making it hard to fall asleep.

(13) Use Sleep Fragrances

Specific smells at nighttime can help you sleep. The main scents that people use for this are:

- Lavender

- Chamomile

- Bergamot

- Jasmine

- Rose

The _Wall street Journal_[14] wrote on the use of lavender in particular as a way to fall asleep faster. Studies have shown that it can slow down your heart rate and decrease your blood pressure.

People react differently to smells. The key is to establish a ritual around the smells and sleep. In addition, you should choose smells that are relaxing and not ones that are too strong.

(14) Dust Your Room

The human skin is continually shedding. Most of the dust in our houses comes from our skin. It is important to ensure the bedroom is dusted and vacuumed. This helps keep the dust mite population at a minimum which helps with allergies. It keeps that dust out of the air and out of your lungs at night.

---

[14]http://www.powerlists.org/avdc

(15) Decorate Your Room With Calming Colors

This tip supports the idea that your room should be a relaxing place that is calming in every way possible. That means you should use wallpaper or paint that is calming to you. Hospitals use this trick to keep people calm. By using off-white or pastels, patients can be kept in a calm state which puts them in a better mood to receive treatment of their medical conditions.

In the same way, your bedroom should not use brilliant colors or splashy eye catching paintings. Rather, it should just be cozy and calm. This might seem as though it is going too far. However, the problems with sleep may be best resolved when combining many small actions to get better and more sleep.

(16) Use Flashlights in the Middle of the Night

When you wake up in the middle in the night needing to go to the bathroom, you might be tempted to turn on the lights. However, turning on the lights will reduce the quantity of melatonin in the system and wake you up.

The trick for getting around this is using flashlights instead of turning on the main lights. In our house, we use motion detecting flashlights. They turn on only when it is night time and when they detect motion. This means we will maximize the amount of melatonin in our system during the night even when going to the toilet.

Using motion detecting LED flashlights requires less electricity, and the children aren't scared to walk out of their rooms in the dark. They know that the flashlights will turn on and guide their way to the bathroom. Sometimes, a simple solution like this makes it easy to sleep well even when waking up in the middle of the night.

(17) Use Bright Lights in the Morning

When morning comes, your body needs to know it is time to wake up. In the ancient world, the sun served this purpose. It may work for you. Exposing yourself to sunlight or bright artificial lights early in the morning may do the trick of getting your body used to waking up at a specific time. This practice may become a ritual you can maintain and therefore have a better flow of moving from nighttime into daytime.

(18) Don't Ignore Pain

The National Sleep Foundation in the US conducted a survey[15] that showed "21 percent reported chronic pain and 36 percent reported acute pain in the past week." The pain that people experience during the day doesn't necessarily go away at night. This pain makes it harder to fall asleep. In addition, it is much more difficult to sleep when in pain.

The solution is to treat your physical pain. Ignoring pain may impact your sleep. That shortage of sleep will come with its own set of consequences. It is better to focus on one issue at a time. If your pain is hurting your sleep, you should focus on fixing this issue as a key way of getting better sleep.

(19) Don't Take Catnaps

We have heard about how power napping can help when we are tired throughout the day. This may be true. However, a nap during the day can wreak havoc on your sleep in the evening.

---

[15]http://www.powerlists.org/ktmo

Falling asleep requires being tired enough to enter the sleep cycle. You can undermine your ability to sleep at night if you take naps throughout the day.

By cutting out naps, you will find it is easier to fall asleep at night. However, as a result you may be more tired during the daytime. Whatever the case, sleeping well at night outweighs the importance of being tired during the day. Better and more regular sleep at night will solve your daytime sleepiness in the long run.

(20) Keep the Bed for Sleeping

This one should make sense without too much thought. However, it is an issue for many people. You want your bed to be associated with sleep. The worst thing you can do in your bed is anything that isn't sleep.

For example, doing work or other activities on your laptop will make you associate the bed with non-sleep related activities and keep you awake.

This trick is hard to implement if you are a student and have one room in a dorm. You will study and work in the room where your bed is located. A good solution is to go somewhere else to do your homework, like the library. The goal is to have your bed associated with sleep.

The bed may also be used for intimate activities, and that is just fine. However, no activities should involve work or school or anything that isn't sleep. An exception to the rule is if you read books at night. Even reading is better done away from the bed. When you get tired, head to your bed.

(21) Don't Read From a Light Emitting Device

It is important to note that you shouldn't be reading on a device that is shooting light at you. That means that an iPad or tablet or phone is a bad idea on the reading front. Instead, use a normal book or turn off the backlight on your Kindle so it isn't shooting light into your eyes.

(22) Keep Your Pets Out of Your Bed

Although it's cozy to have your cat or dog in your bed with you, you should keep pets out of your bed, especially if you are having trouble sleeping. The problem is that the dog or cat will not hold still at night. Rather, they will be moving and flipping their tail. You don't want to be awakened or have your sleep disturbed during the night. So, do yourself a favor and let the pets sleep in their own beds.

(23) Ensure Your House is Secure

Many people fear that intruders will break into their house. They are sensitive to sounds in the middle of the night. The best solution is to secure your house. Make sure you have a security system turned on during the night.

Whether or not your fear is reasonable isn't the issue. Rather, if you are afraid of something happening, you won't be able to sleep. The price of securing your house is nothing when compared to going years without a good night's sleep because of fear.

(24) Exercise

Twenty to thirty minutes of training each day can make a difference in the quality of sleep and the ease at which you fall asleep. Your exercise should be done five hours or more before bed; if the exercise is completed too close to bedtime it can keep you awake.

(25) Ensure Mattress and Pillows Are Comfortable

A surefire way of not getting a good night sleep is to sleep on a mattress that doesn't provide support. Many quality mattresses have a lifespan of a decade. However, people continue to use them long beyond this point. The consequence is losing the support that the mattress provides.

Don't use a pillow that is too large or too small. Be sure the pillow provides support. The easiest way to know whether your pillow or mattress is creating problems for you is to see if you regularly experience back or neck pain in the morning. Ensuring your neck and back are getting the support they need will enable you to:

- Fall asleep quicker

- Be better rested in the morning

(26) Track Your Sleep

I am a huge advocate of tracking your sleep since I love using lists and tracking different aspects of my life. You should keep a journal of how much sleep you are getting.

The process of tracking anything in your life always triggers change. You can find more on the power of lists in my book *Achieve Your Goals Now With PowerLists*™[16] .

When you see your lack of sleep on a piece of paper daily, it is hard not to take it seriously. The same is true with money, food, exercise, and sleep.

Your list need not be fancy. Just include the date in one column and the amount of sleep in the other. Sometimes it is hard to know when you fell asleep. For all intents and purposes, you can start the time when you go to bed and turn off the lights and remove all sound.

Other tricks will focus on how to go from lights off to falling asleep. The first step is to avoid watching TV or using your cell phone.

---

[16]http://www.powerlists.org/xt4x

(27) Quit Using Your Sunglasses

During daytime hours, many people wear sunglasses to block out sunlight or for fashion. However, if you have sleep issues, you should experience as much sunlight as possible for your eyes. This connects back to the internal rhythm of day and night that your body is keeping track of. We discussed keeping it dark at night. It is also important to get daylight during the day since it plays a major role in making sure your body knows it is time to be awake.

The body needs to receive signals when it is day and when it is night. Like setting a clock, you can train your body to keep track of when it is time to wake up and when it is time to sleep. By removing your sunglasses during the day, it won't just wake you up. It will prepare your body for the coming of night time.

(28) Spend Time Outside During the Day

Another trick to getting more sunlight is to be where it is shining. That is outside. We spend much time cooped up in our houses and offices with artificial lights and blue screens from our phones, computers and TVs.

It is essential to break out of the cycle of having the same level and type of light in our eyes all day long regardless of the time. The best way to do this is to get as much sunlight as we can during the day. That helps to program our bodies to know when it is daytime.

(29) Try to Stay Awake

"Keep your eyes wide open, repeat to yourself 'I will not sleep.' The brain doesn't process negatives well, so inter-prets this as an instruction to sleep and eye muscles tire quickly as sleep creeps up." - Julie Hirst. _worklifebalancecentre.org_[17] .

This may appear counterintuitive. However, by telling your-self that you will not go to sleep, you trick the brain into do-ing the opposite. Many times when you tell yourself to sleep and focus on sleeping, you end up not sleeping. The trick to getting you to sleep in no time may be to try the opposite.

(30) Create a Trigger

This is a more advanced technique. We are creatures of habit and we can create triggers with our attempts to go to

---

[17]http://www.powerlists.org/h48a

sleep. For example, you might choose the trigger of rubbing your head as you fall asleep. This then becomes associated with falling asleep.

Whenever you are having a difficult time getting to sleep, you rub your head in the same way. That trigger signals your brain, informing you it is time to sleep. That is what you do right before falling asleep.

(31) Decide on How Much Sleep You Will Get

When trying to get more sleep, you need to decide in advance how much sleep you will get. Like diets and TV consumption, not monitoring your intake means you will move in a negative direction. This is why you must decide up front how much sleep you plan to get.

Even if you cannot fall asleep, you should count the hours you will try to sleep. That should reduce the stress of knowing you still haven't fallen asleep; it doesn't matter if you went to bed at 10 pm.

I recommend you choose a time between seven and nine hours for starters and see if you are rested after that much sleep. If you aren't rested, then you can increase that amount of time. At the same time, if you are waking up early, you may try going to bed later to ensure you wake up as planned.

(32) Keep a Sleep Journal

We discussed tracking the quantity of sleep in a log. However, another trick is to write what tricks you used to fall asleep and how successful they were. After you have a few weeks of data in your sleep journal, you need to change what you are doing based upon what you have learned.

The hard part is that changes can take days to have an impact. When we are trying multiple tricks at once, it may be hard to identify what is helping. However, we don't want to take a year to figure out what is the most important trick for getting you to sleep. Rather, we can try multiple tricks at the same time.

When we find combining these tricks works for us, we can go with that and see if the sleep is good or not. Try creating a checklist of the tricks that work best for you and ensure you practice these tricks daily.

Even if only one or two tricks work, it doesn't matter since the tricks calm us. Their positive impact may not be noticeable at a conscious level. Things can work for us and it may be difficult to see that our REM sleep is better when we keep the room quiet and refrain from eating snacks before bed.

(33) Don't Count the Hours Left to Sleep

Sticking to a schedule and getting in and out of bed at the right times will help you avoid calculating sleep quantities. This practice is guaranteed to decrease stress and produce more sleep.

We need to relax and not try to solve math problems. The worst part of constantly performing calculations is that sleep decreases and stress increases.

Counting sheep can help. The issue is whether the counting or the sheep is a stress point. The main idea is for your mind to fade into the background as you count sheep. It takes your mind off more stressful.

Research has shown that for some people counting sheep is too boring. When bored, our minds move to something more engaging. The problem is that thing that is more engaging may be more stressful.

So, simple math-like counting is fine, but stay away from doing complex math and calculations that are stressful. Just be content with the fact that you are getting to bed on time and will still get rest even if you aren't sleeping. You are training yourself for the routine of sleep.

Oxford researchers[18] found that picturing relaxing images worked better than counting sheep. The images were engaging enough to keep people's minds off the worries of the day. So, just envision a nice, relaxing beach scene or a waterfall in the forest.

(34) Avoid Shift Work

Night shift work may sometimes seem like a good deal. Many companies pay higher salaries or expect less work if you do the non-day shifts. However, it isn't free. Your body pays a price. The internal clock, as discussed earlier, doesn't adjust well.

In addition, the body's response to light and darkness is

---

[18]http://www.powerlists.org/ysxv

thrown off kilter when being forced to stay awake at night and sleep during the day. To ensure you are getting enough sleep, it is best not to agree to work these off shifts.

(35) Don't Sleep in Late

It can be tempting for a person to sleep in if they are sleep deprived. The problem is that this creates additional issues. If you are waking up much later, you will not be tired until even later. Instead, set your alarm and wake up as planned regardless of whether you have to.

Let's assume you are tired from the night before. That extra tiredness will move into the next day and make it easier to fall asleep at the dedicated time. This is better than sleeping in and not being tired the next night when you wish to sleep.

The key here is that we are trying to set up a sleep schedule and hold to it. That schedule will fail if the wake-up time or go-to-sleep time is changed. We can condition our bodies for these two times.

It is important not to sabotage the routine. The weekend is when most people go to bed late and sleep in late. This is fine if we are making the change by an hour. However, it is unwise to allow yourself to vary from your schedule by more than one hour.

(36) Set an Alarm for Sleeping

Habits are key to changing your life, which is why I wrote a book on them. An effective way to make progress with your sleep is to set up a ritual of what needs to be done to get ready for bed. That ritual should include at least an alarm on your phone to remind you each night to start the bedtime ritual.

When the alarm goes off, you need to drop everything and do the first task on your go-to-sleep bedtime routine. This habit will ensure that you don't forget to do something related to sleep, and it will ensure that you don't something unrelated when it is time to sleep.

Many people use alarms to wake themselves up in the morning. However, using alarms at night to tell you to go to sleep seems odd to many people. It is important to have a reminder when it is time to start getting ready for sleep.

For most people, the time we wake up is set based upon getting ready for work or school. That time is rigid for most of us. However, the night before is less structured. We don't have to hurry and go to bed. Sleep can be put off until later.

The problem is that the consequences for that choice aren't doled out until the next day. Daily sleep deprivation makes us experience life as though we are in a hazy cloud. We adjust to this sensation and assume it is normal. When something that is sucking the life from us becomes normal, we are in serious trouble.

One of the tricks for dealing with this is to ensure that you go to bed at the same time each night. This should be done when your alarm goes off and you start the evening bedtime ritual.

(37) Finding Pressure Points

Several areas on the body work as triggers for sleep. I remember using the spot right between the eyebrows on one of my children as a key pressure point when trying to get them to fall asleep. You rub your fingers in a circle while applying pressure.

It can take 30 seconds to a minute to get results with this

method; you can try the same pressure spot on yourself and hold and press for 30 seconds at a time. Other pressure spots can be tried, but this one on your forehead may be the best of them all.

(38) Change Rooms When Unable to Sleep

Many times when we are cannot fall asleep, we will do another activity. This might include work, TV or social media. Whatever the case, make sure you switch rooms with that activity.

Ideally, the activity could be something calming with no screens shooting light at our eyes. Then, we can continue that activity until we are tired and ready to return to bed. It will not help our problem if we roll around in bed for hours. An even worse idea is working in bed.

Studies have shown that being anxious about sleeping and remaining in your bed is a trigger for insomnia. So, it is a better choice to switch rooms and do something else until you feel tired and want to try sleeping again. This will give you something else to think about and maybe even accomplish while away from your bed.

(39) No Sounds at Night

One sure fire way to make sleeping difficult is to be in a noisy environment when you are trying to sleep. Depending upon who is in your family or who your neighbors are, it can be hard to maintain silence. Sounds usually disturb the falling asleep process.

You may have issues with neighbors playing loud music or sounds from the street. That can be impossible to control. A possible solution is to wear ear plugs when you sleep. They are cheap and block out most of the sound.

(40) Set Your Cell Phone on Silent Mode

Most cell phones today have a silent mode. That mode is important when trying to get to sleep. People assume that if they put their phone on vibrate or turn the volume down that this should solve the problem. That is incorrect because vibrate mode still creates sounds. Even in silent mode the screen will light up disturbing sleep both by creating light and tempting us to check it.

Even with the *do not disturb* mode, you can have a list that allows friends or family to get through. You can set the phone to only allow a call through after they have tried twice previously. The goal isn't to ignore the rest of the world in case of a crisis. Rather, you should protect and defend your sleep and ensure that your devices do not create sleeping problems.

(41) Make Your Bed in the Morning

People who make their beds in the morning are 19% more likely to have reported getting a good night's sleep. This may be because the bedroom is clean and organized. In addition, it may be connected to having a routine around the bedroom where you inform yourself at a deep level that morning has come. When you get into bed in the evening, the bed is already made.

(42) Don't Do Stressful Chores Before Bedtime

You may be tempted to do tasks like paying bills or other chores like dishes or mowing your yard before bedtime. This is a bad idea. All activities before bed need to be calming activities. The worst activities to do before bed are ones that are stressful. So, do only calming activities that you enjoy before going to bed.

(43) Don't Do Time Calculations

You might do calculations of how much sleep you will get if you could fall asleep now. Those calculations make you nervous about not getting enough sleep even if you fall asleep immediately. If you don't know the time, you won't be distracted by it.

(44) Arrange to Sleep at the Same Time as Your Partner

If you have a partner you share your bed with, going to bed at the same time will help on multiple fronts. Here are just a few:

- You won't be kept awake by the lights being.

- You won't be awakened when they come to bed.

- You won't hear the sounds they make as they walk around the house or watch TV.

- They can hold you accountable for going to bed as planned at a specific time.

This method doesn't work if you and your partner wake up at different times or start work at different times. Having a common bedtime is a great way to make a habit out of it. It also ensures you both are getting enough sleep.

(45) Don't Look at the Clock in the Middle of the Night

Maybe after falling asleep, wake up in the middle of the night and wonder what time it is. It is a bad idea to check the time. The first problem is your clock shining an LED light in the night. You need to remove that light from your room and return to complete darkness.

Second, looking at the clock can destabilize your emotional calmness. If you realize that it is early, you may worry whether you will fall asleep again. If it is late and you have an hour left to sleep, you may worry whether it is worth sleeping more.

You won't trigger any nervous emotions in the middle of the night if you refuse to look at the clock. You are better off ignoring the temptation and allowing your emotions to stay in order. You were already sleeping and can return to sleep regardless of how much or how little remains.

(46) Focus on Gratitude

Another trick that works is focusing on gratitude. This is a powerful technique for reducing stress and increasing overall happiness. However, the impact of lower stress and higher happiness levels right before bed are what you need when you are finding it difficult to sleep.

(47) Use Your Phone, Not a Standard Digital Clock

Until a few years ago, I used a red letter glowing standard alarm clock. That was a huge mistake. The problem is that it adds light to the room. In addition, it isn't capable of setting alarms to for different sleep schedules for different days.

I studied the impact of light on sleep and put a piece of cardboard over the clock to block the light. I mentioned this to a co-worker, who asked why I wasn't using my cell phone. I didn't have a good answer, and that was the end of using a digital clock for me.

Your smartphone can be programmed to ring on specific days and can even use vibrations and increasing volume levels to make your morning much smoother. The light on the cell phone can be turned off and still have the positive effect of you knowing that the alarm is set.

Many times I have turned off my standard alarm clock without turning it on again for the next night. Now, the only time I sleep in is when the battery has died on my cell phone or I forgot to turn the alarms back on after a vacation.

(48) Stretch Before Bed

Research has shown that stretching can help with your sleep issues. So, by stretching 30 minutes a day you may decrease sleep problems. This study showed a 30% reduction in people struggling with sleep.

(49) Use a Light Therapy Box

During winter days when there is little sun, your body can lose track of when it is day and when it is night. One way to help this is to use a Light Therapy Box which simulates the light that comes from the sun. The goal is to train your body to see it is daytime even when there is little sunlight during the day.

(50) Create a To-do List

By creating a to-do list in writing prior to sleeping, you give yourself permission to not create one while trying to sleep. This method works because the one thing we don't want is stress and worry when we are trying to sleep. We want as little emotion as possible.

By writing all the things we need to remember to do, we give ourselves permission to not worry about those things. We won't forget them since all we have to do is read the list the next day.

What's interesting about this technique is that it doesn't matter whether we do the things on the list. The knowledge they have been written plays a trick on the brain. We realize that we have it recorded and are free to get sleep.

(51) Remove Bright Light Bulbs From Your Bedroom

When trying to sleep at night, the last thing you see shouldn't be a bright light. An easy solution for this is to remove bright light bulbs from your bedroom. This is true if you plan to read or do any other relaxing activity in your bedroom.

Low watt bulbs for your bedroom can help your body build up melatonin. This tip is cheap to implement and can get your sleep routine off to a good start. You enter your bedroom and are greeted by a rather dim light bulb. This trains your brain to know you are heading to bed and it is nighttime.

(52) Review the Day in Detail

A good way to get your mind in a state that will help you fall asleep is to review every event of the day in detail. You start at the beginning of the day and work your way through the day remembering everything you did. This method is similar to counting sheep since it is not very exciting and should slow your thoughts down.

This method isn't so effective if your day was exciting or stressful because instead of slowing your mind down, it will speed it up. It can make you nervous and think about the things you need to remember. So, if you try this method, make sure you choose a day that wasn't exciting.

(53) Make Preparations for Tomorrow

When trying to not stress before bed, you can decrease your stress by creating a plan for the next day. This may include getting everything ready for the morning. In addition, you can choose your clothes or prepare your lunch.

By doing preparation the night before, there are fewer things to worry or think about when you go to sleep. You can sleep knowing everything is ready and in place. Now, your mind is clear to focus on more relaxing themes.

(54) Try White Noise

Some people find that some sounds help them fall asleep. If you are in this category, you may use an app that produces white noise or any sound or music that doesn't distract you from falling asleep.

White noise can include the sounds of:

- Rain

- Wind

- The ocean

- Static

- Anything that doesn't grab your attention

The goal is to relax the mind and brain making it easier to fall asleep. Even something as simple as a clock ticking will serve this trick. Other sounds from your smartphone or computer may work well for you including the following: the beach (water and birds), forest (wind and birds), river (flowing water), or falling rain.

(55) Avoid Caffeine After Lunch

I know how tempting it is to drink a coffee or tea after dinner or right before bed. The problem is that caffeine is a stimulant and will make it harder for you to sleep. Even a single cup of coffee during the day will impact your sleep. I am not saying you should cut out all coffee.

The benefits of drinking coffee far outweigh the downside. However, keep your consumption before lunch time. You may put a cap on how much coffee you consume (between two and three cups per day max). That will give your body time to process the caffeine, but not build an addiction to the coffee.

If you find the other tricks in this book don't work, you should reduce yourself to no caffeine. The goal is to figure out what will get your sleeping in order. When we find that different methods still aren't working for us, it is time for us to take extraordinary measures to get the results we need.

(56) Don't Drink Alcohol Before Bed

This one is even tougher than the caffeine since most people don't drink until later in the evening. In addition, alcohol is a depressant which makes you tired. Don't let that fool you. Alcohol will make your sleep less restful and will leave you tired the next day. The reason for this is that it makes it harder for you to have deep sleep and REM sleep. You will be tired the following day if you are deprived of REM sleep.

I am not saying you should cut out all drinking although you should decrease consumption if you are having an issue getting enough sleep and feeling rested. Sleep is a high priority item that will impact your overall experience of life. So, make the sacrifices necessary to stabilize sleep.

(57) Eat Healthier Food

There is a strong relationship between the food you eat and the quality of sleep you can expect. You should avoid spicy foods and junk foods if you are struggling with the quality and quantity of sleep.

Many of these tricks involve living a healthier lifestyle. By living healthier, you are rewarded with falling asleep quicker, higher quality of sleep, and feeling well rested the next day. You will find great willpower and the ability to keep up with the healthy choices.

(58) Use Separate Blankets if Sharing a Bed

Living in Norway means that each person in a bed has their own eiderdown comforter. That prevents the stealing of blankets in the middle of the night. When visiting the United States and other countries that use normal blankets, my wife and I split the blankets.

The issue is that the tug-of-war in the night can wake you from your sleep. Your top goal is to have as few disturbances as possible. If you are fighting over a blanket all night long, it will be difficult to get a good rest.

The solution is simple to implement. Just ensure that each person has their own comforter or blanket. The other advantage is that it prevents one person from freezing in the middle of the night to discover the other person is wrapped in the shared blanket.

I appreciate that you can move the blanket around to control temperature throughout the night. After moving to Norway, I discovered the superior advantage of these comforters over standard sheets used in the United States. They aren't only more comfortable; they give you a much better night's sleep.

(59) Keep the Baby in a Different Room and Split the Night Into Shifts

This was another issue my wife and I had to learn the hard way. We knew that it was recommended to not have the baby sleep in the bed with us, though we didn't understand just how much a baby can interfere with normal sleeping patterns.

After a few nights in which none of us were getting any sleep, we moved the baby to the other room. That meant that we weren't hearing the baby's sounds all night long. The crying came through the walls, but not the sounds of normal movement and sleeping.

Another trick is splitting the night between you and your partner to allow sleep when it isn't your shift. As this book discusses in the section on sleep cycles, we want to allow a full cycle to complete without disturbances.

If everyone is caring for the baby all night long, the result is no one gets undisturbed cycles of sleep. That's why it is a much better option to split the night in two shifts. Each person gets a four to six hour block of time where they don't have to watch or hear the baby.

(60) Avoid Sugary Drinks

It can be difficult to sleep if you digest sugar right before bedtime. Sugary drinks create insulin spikes. In fact, you shouldn't be drinking anything for two hours before going to bed. . It is best to drink only water, and drink that earlier in the evening..

(61) Fix Your Work/Family Conflicts

A recent study[19] in *Sleep Health Journal* found that "workers who participated in an intervention aimed at reducing conflict between work and familial responsibilities slept an hour more each week and reported greater sleep sufficiency than those who did not participate in the intervention." The role of conflict in our life comes at a price.

---

[19]http://www.powerlists.org/r9po

We need to work hard to ensure our work and home lives have as little conflict as possible if we want to get better sleep. Even an hour a week of sleep loss makes a difference. The main issue here is stress. It is harder to fall asleep while replaying conflicts in the mind. A better solution is to resolve these issues.

(62) Stop Snoring

Snoring has a negative impact on your ability to sleep well through the night. There are several causes of snoring and treatments. For me, losing weight meant the end of snoring. After dropping 37 pounds (17 kg), I quit snoring altogether.

Another trick is to fasten a tennis ball to the back of a t-shirt and wear that to bed. Then, if you are tempted to sleep on your back, the tennis ball will poke you and prevent you from doing this. Sleeping on your side opens your airways and prevents you from snoring.

Another issue is colds and allergies. A stopped up nose and dripping in the throat triggers snoring. This relates to the overall impact of staying healthy. The healthier you are, the better sleep you get, which makes you even healthier.

If you have allergies, you should talk to your doctor regarding solutions. Your sleep is worth taking snoring seriously and you shouldn't let your allergies prevent you from getting proper sleep. My allergy to dust mites meant having my nose filled during the night. After getting allergy medication, this problem went away and I have slept much better.

Realize that your partner's snoring will negatively impact your sleep. This can be the case even if you feel like you sleep through their snoring. During specific stages of your sleep cycle you are more sensitive to surrounding sounds.

So, if this problem is serious, you may need to sleep in a different room. Another option is to ensure that you go to sleep before they do. That will give you a head start before they snore.

(63) Sleep in a Better Position

Although it may seem like it doesn't matter which position you sleep in, it matters for getting a better night's sleep. The ideal position for sleep is on your back. The downside of this position is that it can lead to snoring. However, that may be a reasonable price to pay if you are having issues with sleep deprivation.

Sleeping on your belly is the worst position. A middle position is that of sleeping on your side. This position has its benefits if you are using the correct pillow to keep your spine in proper alignment. I like the side position best. However, if I lose my pillow during the night, I pay for this position with pain in the neck and back the next morning.

(64) No Large Meals Before Bed

You may experience problems with sleeping well if you are eating large meals two to three hours prior to going to bed. A better trick is to have small snacks if you get hungry before bed. That will help you deal with the hunger without inhibiting your sleep.

Here are a few snacks that can be great when trying to sleep:

- A banana

- Warm milk

- Turkey meat

- Cereal

- Yogurt

The key here is that the food isn't heavy and will fill your hunger needs without hurting your ability to sleep.

(65) 4-7-8 Breathing Trick

Controlling your breathing is a common trick used to fall asleep. It is simple and yet effective. The pattern of breathing looks like this:

- Breathe in through your nose for four seconds

- Hold your breath for seven seconds

- Exhale through your mouth for eight seconds

This breathing method is effective whenever you wish to calm down. The result is like a sedative. This is why this method is so effective for falling asleep.

The problem it solves is under-breathing. When we are stressed we get too little oxygen and our breathing is too rapid.

(66) Don't Smoke Before Bed

Cigarettes have nicotine, which is a stimulant. That serves to wake you up. If you want to get better sleep, consider smoking earlier in the day. Unlike drinking coffee, there are no health benefits to smoking, only losses.

You should work to cut smoking out of your daily routine; however, this book isn't about health habits. Rather, it is focused on doable changes you can make to improve your sleep. Try to decrease the quantity of cigarettes you smoke and ensure they are being smoked early in the day; before lunch, if possible.

(67) Get Your Stress and Worries Under Control

There is nothing worse than trying to sleep while you are focused on all of the stress and worries of the past day or the next day. Dealing with stress is a huge area in its own right which is worth solving if it is a problem.

When you allow yourself to live in a state of constant stress, it comes at a price of worse sleep. This lack of sleep increases the amount of stress and decreases your ability to cope with that stress. Thus, the cycle goes round and round with stress impacting sleep and your poor sleep increasing your stress. This is why I argue that if you are dealing with stress, you should get it under control.

(68) Ensure Proper Ventilation

Many people underestimate the importance of proper ventilation and the role it plays on the air quality in your bedroom. The air in your room should be fresh. This may mean installing better ventilation or opening a window.

Using air conditioning can help with this. If you find that the room is too dry, a humidifier will help. If it is too humid, a dehumidifier may do the trick.

You need to experiment with the air in your room. If you want to maximize the quality of your sleep, controlling the quality of the air is a perfect way to do this.

(69) Keep the Room Cool

The temperature of your bedroom can make a big difference. You don't want to be freezing at night, but boiling will also be a problem. The ideal temperature is between 60 and 67F (16 - 20C).

This temperature zone is a perfect range for getting the best possible quality of sleep. For many people this temperature range is too cold. However, with blankets, you will sleep fine.

(70) Wear Minimal Clothing

It's tempting to wear wool to bed at night. However, if you are sweating during the night in your sleep, you won't find it to be so restful. A better option is to wear as little clothing as possible. Your sheets and blankets should provide enough warmth and you should keep the room temperature cool.

One way to know whether you are sleeping with too much clothing on is to see if you are sweating when you wake up in the middle of the night. If so, you need to adjust what you are wearing to bed. Most pajamas are lightweight and made of cotton or other material suited for sleeping.

There is another advantage with pajamas or any clothes you only wear when going to bed. They establish a ritual and clothing that is associated with sleeping. It is like putting on a night cap, telling your brain it is time to sleep now. These cues can be powerful in creating an entire series of triggers to make you sleepy.

Make sure these clothes are only worn when you will sleep. The next morning, you should change out of your clothes before leaving your room. The reason is that these clothes will be associated with breakfast, coffee, checking e-mail and such if you don't keep them only for your bedroom.

(71) Visualize Yourself in a Happy Place

Visualization can be a powerful tool to put your mind in the right state to get sleep. Imagine yourself in a calm and relaxing place and let your brain relax there. This might be in the forest or at the beach as you watch the waves roll in.

The key to this is that you aren't thinking about trying to sleep, but rather are allowing the environment within the visualization to do the work for you. Just make sure the location isn't exciting. You want to go to sleep, not wake up.

(72) Focus on the Sensations of Your Body

Over thinking can make it difficult to fall asleep. A great trick for stopping yourself from over thinking is to stop everything and try to feel the sensations of the different parts of your body. That sets the focus on the here and now. This method is found within the practice of mindfulness or living in the moment.

Stop your mind from moving away to the past or the future and just focus on what your body is feeling right here and now. When done correctly, it is much easier to fall asleep since you are preventing or blocking your mind from focusing on themes that keep you awake.

Much of your stress is associated with memories of the past or anxiety for the future. Unless you are in this moment experiencing pain, this method can protect you from the stress of the past or future.

(73) Dim the Light

As we have discussed earlier, avoiding computer screens of

any kind is important to sleep. However, lamps that have bright lights that can create problems for you. You sleep best when your body knows it is nighttime. That will happen if you don't expose yourself to bright lights.

One solution is to have dimmers on lights. As the night goes on, you can hit the dimmer switch on the lamps. It will prepare you for sleep. If you can't dim the lights in your house, you will want to turn them off after a specific time. You need to give your body time to adjust to the idea it is time to get sleep.

(74) Use Cognitive Behavioral Therapy for Insomnia (CBTI)

"CBTI consists of several components that are tailored to the patient's individual presentation. Stimulus control, developed by Richard Bootzin, is a set of instructions that address conditioned arousal." Cognitive Behavioral Therapy for Insomnia (CBTI)[20] , *Stanford Health Care.*

This therapy is an effective way of getting more and better sleep. A trained therapist can look at your individual issues

---

[20]http://www.powerlists.org/fz56

and help tailor a program with special focus in the following areas:

- Stimulus control

- Sleep restriction

- Sleep-interfering arousal/activation

- Foods and substances

- Biological clock

I have explored each of these methods in this book; however, this method is different because you are working with a trained professional who is able to guide you in finding the correct techniques, balance and focus for you. The other advantage is that this therapy uses no drugs to accomplish this goal.

12 - Final Thoughts

In this book we have explored:

- What is sleep

- Stages of sleep

- Signs you aren't getting enough

- Myths about sleep

- Consequences of not getting enough sleep

- The benefits of sleep

- The different sleep problems

- Why we don't sleep more

- Why not use drugs

- Tricks for better sleep

There is one goal here. I want you to get adequate amounts of a higher quality sleep. That is why we took time to explore why you are having problems and what can be done to fix this situation. The most important thing is to try something. Ideally, you would try multiple tricks from this book until you find what works best for you. These methods have been tried, tested, and proven to help people like you get better sleep.

I am not saying that if you follow them all, you will have perfect sleep. Rather, I argue that small improvements in sleep will have huge rewards for you including more and/or improved sleep. Keep in mind that the symptoms of poor sleep often cause you to get worse sleep. This spiral effect needs to be broken. When your sleep ritual is in place, other issues fall away.

I hope this book will help you get superior sleep. If you have other tricks and know of helpful research, let me know. I am always updating my books to make sure they are as comprehensive and up-to-date as possible. We are all in this life together and it makes sense to help each other live it better.

Remember to pick up your Easy Sleep Solutions Cheat Sheet[21] if you haven't already downloaded it. It is great as a checklist to see which tricks you have tried and also is a quick one page refresher of the contents of this book.

---

[21]http://www.powerlists.org/7v84

Thank You

As we reach the end of this book, I want to say thanks for reading this book.

I want to get this information out to as many people as possible. If you found this book helpful, I would greatly appreciate you leaving me a review. This helps others find the book as well.

Disclaimer

This document is geared towards providing exact and reliable information in regards to the topic and issue covered. The publication is sold on the idea that the publisher is not required to render an accounting, officially permitted, or otherwise, qualified services. If advice is necessary, legal, financial, medical or professional, a practiced individual in the profession should be ordered.

This information is not presented by a financial or medical practitioner and is for entertainment, educational and informational purposes only. The content is not intended as a substitute for professional medical advice, diagnosis, or treatment. Always seek the advice of your physician or other qualified health care provider with any questions you may have regarding a medical condition. Never disregard professional medical advice or delay in seeking it because of something you have read.

The information provided herein is stated to be truthful and consistent, in that any liability, in terms of inattention or otherwise, by any usage or abuse of any policies, processes, or directions contained within is the solitary and utter responsibility of the recipient reader. Under no circumstances

DISCLAIMER

will any legal responsibility or blame be held against the publisher for any reparation, damages, or monetary loss due to the information herein, either directly or indirectly.

Last Updated: 11.Nov.2020